SENSUAL SORCERY

Natural beauty and
health recipes

Stella Ralfini

Typeset in ITC New Baskerville

Editing, design, typesetting and publishing by UK Book Publishing

www.ukbookpublishing.com

Photography: © Mary Dimou

Book cover: George Pazalos

ISBN: 978-1-913179-11-3

To celebrate publication of Sensual Sorcery, I have teamed up with respected aromatherapy supplier Soap Kitchen who will send you a **FREE** bottle of Lavender Essential Oil as a bonus. All you have to do is purchase a 100ml bottle of Sweet Almond carrier oil (which you need anyway to make beauty recipes).

Use the code below and your free Lavender Oil will be added to your cart.

The Soap Kitchen stock a vast range of carrier/essential oils, containers and everything else you might need at reasonable cost. Their products are high quality and their service second to none.

Claim your bottle of Lavender oil by using this code in check-out at... *https://www.thesoapkitchen.co.uk*
SENSLAV5

(Kindly note this offer is open to one code use per person. Offer may be withdrawn without notice.)

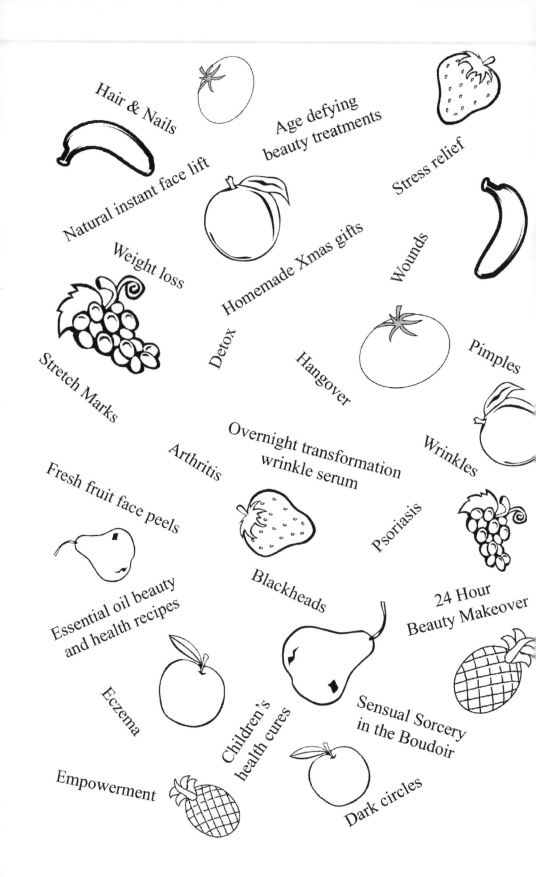

CONTENTS

SENSUAL SORCERY

*'I'm not a woman who needs
to be saved from dragons. I eat
them for breakfast every day.'*

When women see me for the first time they say 'You can't *possibly* be in your seventies, you have the skin of a much younger woman.' I smile, firstly because even I cannot believe how or when I reached this age and secondly because my skin *is* exceptional and I'm proud of it.

Sensual Sorcery will hopefully prove that buying expensive beauty products isn't the answer to holding back wrinkles. We have to start on the inside, be done with junk food (other than occasional naughty treats), eat fruits and vegetables in abundance, drinks lots of water, know which vitamins to take and treat our bodies with respect. Once we find balance with that aspect, beauty automatically shines through.

I might have a glamorous, diva persona, but at heart I'm a hippie who finds nature a source of wonder. I have been making natural beauty/health products for nearly as long as I have been an empowerment teacher and beauty/

health advisor, and in the same way a gourmet chef strives to perfect his recipes, I strive to better my natural beauty creations.

I will include tips passed down by my gran and mum, both of whom had fantastic skin into their eighties, together with beauty tips gathered on travels to far-flung countries across the globe.

Nearly all fruits and vegetables that are beneficial for us on the inside, serve our skin equally well. This does not perhaps apply to beetroot since we'd look pretty stupid walking around with a purple face. However, from now on when you munch on a carrot, bite into a banana, take a mouthful of avocado, tomato, apple, grapefruit, apricot or peach, know that these and many more fruits will become your besties as we work together through this book.

Same thing applies to thyme, rosemary, mint, turmeric, basil, star anise and numerous other herbs. Apart from their use to season dishes, we will use these treasures to season our hair, skin and nails.

Maybe at this point you are just starting out on the natural homemade beauty trail but I promise that within no time, you will become such an expert in the craft, you'll be whipping up Coconut Soufflé Body Cream and Strawberry-Vanilla Mousse Exfoliator with the ease of whipping an egg.

Do not be rigid. Use my recipes as a guideline. Push yourself to experiment with different carrier oils and essential oils. As your knowledge grows, decrease or increase ingredients given in my recipes until you find what works best for your skin type and allow the alchemist inside you to come out to play.

While the recipes in this book are listed in Alphabetical order, many use a number of ingredients which cross over and lend a hand with others. So for example, honey, avocado and egg crop up numerous times in different recipes.

I did not devise Sensual Sorcery as a book to read from start to finish but as something to dip into as the mood takes. Therefore, if you're thinking about having a detox day or one where you wish to concentrate on wrinkles, eye bags or hair, you can go straight to that page and take your pick from a smorgasbord of suggestions.

Rather than scratch your head wondering what to make, another way to use this book is to open it at random and make suggested recipe(s) on that page. You will often find that your random pick is exactly what your face, body or health needs - and it's a fun approach to encourage you to try out ideas you might otherwise overlook.

I hope you find Sensual Sorcery informative, recipes easy to make and are thrilled with the results. These were my priorities when compiling this book.

I think the time has arrived to get started with the basics, don't you? Turn the page and we will begin...

INDEX OF MY FAVOURITE CARRIER AND ESSENTIAL OILS

The list of carrier oils and essential oils that can be incorporated in natural homemade products is vast, so I am sticking with 5 carrier oils for this book. Having understood their uses, you might decide a couple of carrier oils are enough at this stage - which is fine. Essential oils are a different ball game. I use around 30 since I make so many different products. For you, I have chosen six that represent starter kit *musts* for any self-respecting beauty diva.

My Five Favourite Carrier Oils:
Sweet almond oil. Sweet almond oil is made with edible almonds and is so mild and hypoallergenic that it is often used on baby skin. It is endowed with highly potent antioxidant vitamin E which protects skin from UV radiation damage and oxidative stress. It can be used safely on sensitive skin since it rarely causes allergic reactions.

Coconut oil is a brilliant source of vitamins A, C and E and is a super oil for facial massage since it's incredibly moisturizing. It reduces appearance of wrinkles, brings elasticity back to skin and gives it a healthy glow. Coconut oil is widely used in face, body and hair beauty products but is of particular value when used in anti-wrinkle facial products since it hardens when kept in the 'fridge and can be applied in tiny amounts to work around the eye around.

Jojoba oil is light in texture, doesn't feel greasy on your skin and penetrates deep into pores, tightening them whilst hydrating the skin at the same time. Full of healthy antioxidants and valuable Vit E, it rarely produces allergic reaction so is another winner.

Apricot Kernel oil is pressed from the kernels of the Prunus armeniaca apricot. It is rich in Vitamin K (which is believed to reduce dark circles), Vitamin E (another super skin food), Vitamin C and omega fatty acids. Since it is easily absorbed by the skin it is often used for massage purposes and has such nourishing qualities, is used in many beauty recipes.

Argan Oil is a rare and precious oil that is harvested and extracted from the nut of the Argan tree. With its high content of antioxidants, essential fatty acids and Vitamin E, it has the ability to naturally revitalize and hydrate skin. Add to this that it's a powerful UV protector and free-radical neutralizer which rarely causes allergic reaction, and we have another winner.

ESSENTIAL OILS

A few facts before I list six of my favourite essential oils. I'm sure you know this but just in case you didn't, beauty products are one of the least regulated consumer products on the market. It is said that one in six cosmetic products contain chemicals linked to cancer and that only thirteen percent of ingredients used in personal care products are reviewed by an official governing board. This isn't good news since the skin is our largest organ and what goes on the face or body goes in.

With the beauty products we'll make together we will use the wisdom supplied by Mother Nature so as not to further add to the toxic burden we laden our bodies with. This means the essential oils we use should be 100% pure and not blended with any other ingredients or oils. The blended form of essential oil is cheaper but doesn't do the same job so ensure it says '100% pure' on the bottle before you buy.

Essential oils aren't oils in the way you may have perceived them until now and come under the category of 'ethereal' oils. This means that the aromatic compounds found in fruits, herbs, flowers and plants are extracted through lengthy, complicated steam distillation to obtain tiny amounts of the subsequent oils. This is no small task when we consider that one drop of essential rose oil equals around 60 ground rose petals.

Rose essential oil. One of the reasons wrinkles appear with age is due to the drop of collagen production which causes skin to lose its elasticity. Rose oil is a firm favourite because of its ability to turn the clock back when used on a regular basis. Rose oil also has a delicious smell but its properties, qualities and healing powers are monumental. It's antimicrobial, hydrating, tightening benefits make it an excellent choice for use in natural homemade anti-aging beauty products. According to extensive studies carried out by Chinese researchers a few years back, rose oil exhibited one of the strongest bacterial activities compared to many other essential oils. This means it also excels for anyone who suffers with pimples, acne and skin eruptions.

Taken a step further, a few drops of rose essential oil mixed with a teaspoon of carrier oil for massage purposes, helps to ease cramps, fatigue, and relaxes the intestinal muscles, offering fast relief from constipation while helping to maintain a healthy digestive system. It is very easy to massage yourself since concentration should be on the stomach area. I do it whenever I feel bloated and it works a treat.

Frankincense essential oil. Due to my age, Frankincense goes into nearly every beauty recipe I make. Frankincense promotes cell regeneration, strengthens the skin's elasticity and gives skin a healthy, radiant glow. It also protects against liver spots (age spots) which is one of the plights of getting older.

Taken a step further, a few drops of Frankincense oil mixed with a teaspoon of carrier oil, works wonders when used for neck massage since it increases oxygenation of the pituitary gland. This helps to balance mood swings and gives us a more relaxed mind state.

Lavender essential oil. Another absolute must for your starter kit. Lavender oil is beneficial for skin disorders such as acne, psoriasis and other inflammatory conditions. Used regularly it inhibits the bacteria which causes initial infection and over excretion of sebum. Anyone with greasy skin would benefit from Lavender oil as would nervous, anxious personality types.

Lavender oil has highly researched evidence that it is of immense use to counteract migraines, headaches and stress, and due to its effect on the autonomic nervous system is valued as an aid for insomnia. It is also widely used in body massage to combat tense muscles, backache and rheumatism. For you to use it, I recommend mixing a few drops of Lavender oil with a teaspoon of carrier oil and rubbing it behind your ears if you suffer with headaches, rub lower spine area for back ache, or painful joint to ease tense muscles. (When I was recovering from melanoma cancer, my legs stiffened up so I massaged my thighs with lavender oil and it did somewhat release the pain).

Geranium essential oil. Another gem with a myriad of uses. Geranium oil has super astringent qualities and can be used equally well on dry, oily or combination skin. Due to its excellent hemostatic properties, Geranium oil is wonderful for treating eczema, pimple and acne and also for regenerating new skin tissue.

Carrot Seed essential oil. This might be one of the most overlooked essential oils in aromatherapy. Packed with powerful antioxidants, Vits A, K, potassium and magnesium it decreases sun damage from UV exposure, visibly improves skin tone, elasticity, slows down appearance of fine lines and wrinkles and keeps age spots at bay. Carrot seed oil is what we might call a 'reviving' oil. Praised for its ability to stimulate cell growth, it is ideal for those with irritated or mature skin.

Patchouli essential oil. If you're around my age, you might associate Patchouli with hippies, and the 'make love not war' era when it was used profusely in incense sticks. Don't be put off by this. For Patchouli oil to make our list, means I highly value it to address skin issues. As with the other oils listed above it has antioxidant, anti-inflammatory properties, said to be a tissue regenerator and assist growth of skin cells and heal scar tissue. Patchouli oil has an honoured place in Asian medicine and is used to effectively treat dandruff, oily scalp, acne and eczema.

Cautions. Please be sure you do not have allergies to eggs, nuts, milk, cream and whatever else so many have become allergic to in recent years before making recipes that contain them. Also, where uncertain if a particular essential oil might cause allergic reaction, test patch on inner elbow before applying to your face. Pregnant women should seek the advice of their doctor before using essential oils. My health tips should also not be taken as medical advice. If I tell you not to eat bananas and you know they give you constipation but eat them anyway, I will not be held responsible.

AVOCADO BEAUTY TREATMENTS

*'If you want to be happy,
be exactly who you are.'*

Avocado and Carrot Mask to Rebuild Skin Collagen

Mae West famously said 'The only carrots I'm interested in are the carats you find in diamonds.' While I'm fond of that kind of carat myself, I'm also into vegetable carrots big time.

Sometimes when I've been on a long flight, my skin bears witness to the fact. I did on one occasion – having become a carrot fanatic shortly beforehand - ask room service at my hotel to bring me the ingredients for this mask explaining I had an important meeting that afternoon and wanted to look my best. He probably felt like saying 'Use the hotel beauty salon, you stingy cheap-skate.' However, without batting an eyelid he presented me with:

One cooked carrot, a ripe avocado, an egg and a little jug of single cream (the type you put in coffee).

Twirling his moustache, he watched me mush everything together in a bowl while I told him that carrot, avocado and egg fed the skin with Vit A, C, E, beta carotene and antioxidants, that the cream added protein and calcium and the four drops of essential Rose oil (added to mix from the essential oil emergency kit I carry with me everywhere), dealt with fine lines and would encourage a glow. He left none the wiser. I went to my meeting feeling sassily refreshed.

Want to have a go? Just mash 1 (small) cooked carrot with quarter ripe avocado, an egg and one tbs single cream. Keep mashing until you have a smooth paste, add 4 drops essential Rose oil, mix once more then apply over face/neck/chest. To give skin a deeply nourishing treatment, leave mask on for 30 mins before rinsing off with warm water.

Avocado and Honey Facial Mask with Geranium oil

When your skin feels really dry, here's a super nourishing mask.

Blend together quarter ripe **avocado,** 1 tsp **honey,** 1 tsp **Vitamin E oil** and 4 drops essential **Geranium oil**. Together they are an ultra-moisturizing cluster of queen bees. Whip, whip, whip until you have a creamy paste. Using a makeup brush or clean fingers, apply mask over face and neck. Leave on for 20 minutes then rinse off with warm water.

Avocado Eye Mask

If you're in the mood to go the whole hog and reap more benefits from avocado, here's an eye mask to relieve tired eyes which you can simultaneously apply while your face mask is drying. (I know. I'm a slave driver!)

Blend 1/8 of a ripe **avocado**, 1/8 cup of pure **Aloe Vera** gel with 2 drops **Frankincense oil.** Mash to a smooth paste. Using clean fingers, apply to the area under your eyes. Leave on for 20 minutes then wash off with warm water.

Avocado Hair Mask

But hold on a minute, if you've got avocado all over your face, neck and under your eyes, why leave it there when you can give your hair an amazing treat to not only moisturize, revitalize and deal with split ends but give your locks more va va voom?

Half ripe avocado. One egg yolk, 1 tbs coconut oil, 6 drops Rosemary oil.
Mash half ripe avocado. Mix well with one egg yolk, one tbs coconut oil and 6 drops Essential Rosemary oil. Mash into a paste then massage mixture well into scalp and hair. Cover with shower cap. Leave on for 20 minutes then shampoo and condition as normal.

Avocado Hand Mask

No, no, don't worry. You do *not* have to make another mask for your hands. You simply ensure that you have a little of your **Avocado and Honey face mask** left over. Massage a thin layer of avocado mixture into the back of your hands, slip hands into a pair of thin plastic gloves (the type used when we tint our hair). Leave on 15 mins then rinse off with warm water....

If you are now covered from head to fingernails in avocado, well done you. You are going to feel divine when it comes off.

ANISE STAR AND APPLE. TWO SECRET BEAUTIFIERS

'Keep them going. Dreams don't have an expiration date.'

Anise Star Wrinkle Busting Skin Tonic.

The creation of my anise wrinkle busting skin tonic came about at the same time I fell in love with fenugreek many moons ago. **Fenugreek** is an excellent herb where beauty is concerned since not only is it packed with minerals, it is rich in folic acid, vitamin B6, vitamins A and C and niacin. What skin wouldn't want a burst of those wrinkle busters?

The **anise**, with its antiseptic, antibacterial properties add protection against skin outbreaks, the 6 drops of **Rose, Geranium or Frankincense** oil give further help in dealing with wrinkles and the **Rose Water** provides a soothing base.

All you need is: I bottle Rose Water (available in pharmacies and health shops). 1 Star Anise (you can either use 1 Star Anise, crushed into powder or 2 drops star anise essential oil) Half tsp fenugreek powder. 2 drops each of Rose, Geranium and Frankincense oil.

Tip fenugreek powder, star anise and 6 drops essential oil into your Rose Water bottle, close top, give bottle a shake and its ready for use.

You can use your wrinkle busting tonic in two ways. One is straight from the Rose Water bottle in which case you simply pour a little onto a cotton pad and dab face/neck with it. The other is to transfer skin tonic to glass spray bottle and lightly spray face and neck (which I prefer). Whichever route you take, use your tonic straight from the refrigerator.

Exfoliating Apple Sauce Face Mask.

No wonder they say 'an apple a day keeps the doctor away.' Apples aren't just great for health though. They contain Vitamin A,C,E,K and B, are high in fruit acids (think natural face peels) and Niacin Folate and Pantothenic Acid. Oh boy, what more could the skin want than a blast of those…Let's have a look at what we need:

2 tbs **applesauce.** From a jar is fine. I usually buy applesauce made for babies. 1 tsp **ground oats**. 1 tsp **honey.** 1 tsp **lemon, lime and orange juice** (or 1 drop each of **lemon, lime and orange oil)**

Combine all the ingredients in a bowl and apply to face and neck. Leave on for 10 minutes then gently rub skin in circular motions to take off dead skin before rinsing off with warm water. If you're in the mood to give your skin more tender love, follow with this super skin quenching Apple Souffle Face Mask.

Apple Souffle Face Mask *(to deeply nourish skin)*

Quarter jar baby **apple sauce.** 1 tbs **ground oatmeal,** (available at health shops)**.** 1 tbs plain **yoghurt. 6 drops** Frankincense oil. 1 tbs **oat starch** (to thicken).

Blend apple sauce with other ingredients and keep mixing until you have a smooth consistency. Apply to face and neck. Leave on for 20 mins and rinse off with warm water.

Apple/Olive Oil Face Mask.

I used to watch my mum whisk this one up on occasion. Have no idea where she got the recipe or how much it added to her exceptional skin but thought I'd pass it on since it's a great one for women over 60.

Mush half an apple in a dish until it looks like apple sauce. Add 1 tsp of **rose water** and 1 tsp of **olive oil.** Mix ingredients well. Apply to face, neck and around eyes. Leave on 20 mins then rinse off.

You'll have realized by now that most natural recipes are quite messy? They eventually stick to the skin but maybe you could lie back and think about how you're going to spend your lottery win until they dry a little.

ARTHRITIC CONDITION HEALTH SOLUTIONS

'Ponder on the power that creates oak trees from acorns and feel the power you've been given to heal and grow.'

I see that as my age increases, I have the beginnings of arthritis and know it is a condition with which many suffer. When my legs feel particularly stiff, I bite the bullet and dedicate myself to a week of dealing with it in the manner I'm about to suggest.

The glass of raw potato juice last thing at night takes a while to adjust to but like everything else it's a case of mind over matter and it's important to put our health first eh…

Special Veg Soup for Arthritic Conditions

Any vegetables of choice with 1 cup stinging nettles, 1 cup dandelion leaves, 2 tbs licorice powder, (these ingredients are available in most health shops) 2 tbs garlic, 2 tbs turmeric, 1 tsp fresh grated ginger and 1 tsp flaxseeds. Boil cut veg with rest of ingredients in enough water to make three good servings for the week. On these three days I find it best to have a healthy filling lunch and eat this soup in the evening so the cure can carry on working while I sleep.

1 hour before lunch, chew 2/3 juniper berries thoroughly then swallow (juniper berries have been used since ancient times to relieve joint pain, gout, rheumatoid arthritis and nerve, muscle and tendon disorders).

You also need to take 2000ml Cod Liver oil every day. (A 1000ml capsule after breakfast and another 1000ml capsule after lunch). You need 1500ml of Glucosamine Sulphate to be taken 3x a day in 500ml dose capsules after breakfast, lunch and dinner and 1000ml of Vitamin C with your morning dose of Cod Liver oil and Glucosamine Sulphate. They take 6-8 weeks to kick into the system so I suggest that you take them for at least three months.

Half glass raw potato juice (can dilute with water) last thing at night

Notes: Avoid red meat and include the following foods as regularly as possible. Pineapple, red peppers (all kinds), rosemary, oregano, avocado and grapefruit.

Porridge Poultice for Painful Joints. And here we have another recipe, courtesy of my mum, to alleviate throbbing muscles.

All you need to do is boil some porridge in the least amount of water possible to keep it thick. You don't want to scold yourself but this cure needs to be as hot as you can bear to draw out the pain. Slap the porridge in a cloth tea towel, wrap around painful area, leave on until porridge cools then remove. My mum didn't know about essential oils but we do, so to make this cure more potent, you can massage painful area with a few drops of either Peppermint, Lavender or Juniper essential oil before applying poultice.

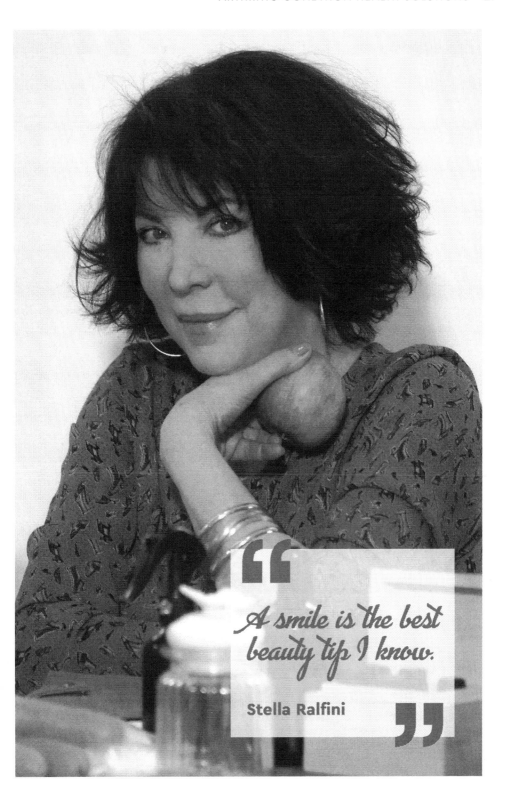

" A smile is the best beauty tip I know.

Stella Ralfini

BANANAS FOR WEIGHT LOSS, HEALTH AND BEAUTY

'When you feel ready to give up remember how many battles you've won. Dust off your armour and rise.'

Already a Hatha and Kundalini yoga teacher, some years back I added Tantra Yoga to my qualifications. Tantra yoga is for couples who want to get closer physically, mentally and spiritually and teaches that honest communication between partners holds the key to better lovemaking. (Should you wish to read more, it's all in my book *Three Faces of Sex*). Tantra certainly taught me how to be more honest. It also taught me heaps about essential oil uses and health.

The Tantra banana detox I am going to share, isn't just a brilliant way to give your health a boost. It helps to shift extra pounds through the use of two simple ingredients. **Bananas** and **Cardamom** pods. Working together, this miraculous duo adjusts the iron, sodium and potassium factors in our body so that our metabolism speeds up and remembers to chew fat up and spit it out instead of hoarding it like a miser.

Breakfast: 1 cup freshly squeezed orange juice with pulp left in. Sweeten with honey if you wish.

After one hour eat two bananas including any strings that stick to them and chew thoroughly. Immediately after the bananas, eat contents of one whole cardamom pod. (The cardamom turns the banana into a liquid which gets to work on the digestive system to speed up metabolism).

Lunch: 2 bananas followed by one whole cardamom pod.
Dinner: 2 bananas followed by one whole cardamom pod.

When thirsty during the day, drink lots of water and 2 more glasses orange/honey juice. If you find the detox makes you constipated, increase cardamom pods to 3 to rectify.

At the end of the night, have a big glass of warm water with lemon and honey.

To carry on body organ cleansing process, the banana detox is followed by a day where we eat fruits for breakfast and a lunch of cooked brown rice with green vegetables, i.e. green beans, courgettes, green peppers, broccoli, cabbage, kale, spinach. Mix turmeric and finely chopped fresh mint into the green vegetables to aid digestion.

Evening snack is a pot of plain yoghurt.

A true yogi could keep this banana detox up for two weeks. I never made it past two days. However, I don't believe in being hard on myself. This is how I managed to get to the fourteenth day finishing line by doing it my way.

1 banana detox day, followed by one brown rice day. The third and fourth day I chose what to eat (obviously no meat, no fried foods, bread, cakes, pastries etc.) Fifth and sixth day was another banana detox and brown rice day. The next two days I chose what to eat then went back to a banana and rice day and so on until I reached fourteen days. Even though I cheated, I did shift some weight and felt energized so you may wish to grit your teeth and give the Tantra detox a go.

Whey Protein Banana Fruit Shake. Due to the fact I'm dedicated to staying in shape, on the whole my weight stays steady. However, I do have a penchant for chocolate; when on holiday make a pig of myself and have occasional weeks when all I want to eat is pizza and French fries. After a few weeks of overindulgence my body balks by not allowing me to fasten my zip, which is when I replace a meal a day with my delicious Whey Protein Banana Fruit Shake. Rather than explain here how to make, it might be easier if you watch me do so on my YouTube channel. It's video 3 in my Sensual Sorcery series with the title 'How to Lose Weight, Healthily, Tastily and Fast.'

Banana masks. From health to beauty, bananas are a must to nourish the skin. Packed with Vitamin C, potassium, Vitamin B6, minerals and antioxidant compounds, they have multiple uses in skin care recipes. Last night was one of those nights when I gave my skin a beauty treat using this magical fruit. My skin today has a lovely, healthy glow thanks to the banana sugar scrub and hydrating face mask I made, so join me and go bananas beautiful all.

Banana Sugar scrub. Mash together one third of a **banana** with one tbs of **demerara sugar** and mix until you have a paste. Apply to your skin using gentle circular motions then rinse off with cool water. As you'll see, your skin will feel smooth and look energised. Let's carry on with step 2.

Hydrating Banana Face Mask: To make this ultra-moisturizing mask, blend quarter of a **banana** with one tablespoon of **honey** until it has a smooth consistency. Using a makeup, pastry brush or your fingers (which may get a little sticky!), apply to your face and neck. Leave on for 20 minutes then rinse off with warm water.

BEAUTY STARTS INSIDE. TREAT YOUR BODY LIKE A TEMPLE

*'If you're not taking chances,
you're going nowhere.'*

Our eyes might be the windows to our souls but they are also the first thing we see in a mirror. Not always a pleasant sight eh…

Dark Circles.

In Alfred Vogel's health manual 'The Nature Doctor'. Vogel, a respected Swiss naturopath, states that dark circles are often symptoms of liver disorders and constipation. To remedy them he suggests drinking lots of carrot juice, taking a daily calcium complex tablet and liver restorer Milk Thistle (available in health shops).

Incorporate different foods into your diet every day that contain high amounts of vitamin C. These can build collagen, which makes your skin look firmer. They can also protect your skin from UV damage that causes wrinkling. Some examples of foods high in Vitamin C include:

Tomatoes. Chili peppers. Mango. Strawberries, Broccoli. Pineapple.

Berries. Use a wide selection of colorful berries regularly. (Strawberry, Raspberry, Blackberries and Blueberries. These contains polyphenols and antioxidants that promote cell regeneration that may reduce the appearance of wrinkles and prevent them.

Herbs to consider: Astragalus – Ayurvedic/Chinese medicine used to strengthen immune system, particularly useful for someone weakened through illness or chronic fatigue syndrome. Also believed to slow growth of cancer cells.

Dandelion. Improves energy levels by detoxifying body.

Ginger. Helps body to release toxins.

Green Tea. Full of antioxidants which prevent disease and cancer. Eliminates toxins and boosts energy levels.

Milk thistle. Cleanses liver, clears out toxins and boosts energy. (Use with dandelion to help metabolism work more efficiently).

If you get dark circles around your eyes, you can minimize them by using raw **potato** in this way. Cut a thin slice of raw potato in two pieces, place under eyes and leave on for 10 minutes. If done on a regular basis, raw potato lightens the skin around your eyes.

For puffy eyes, I came across this gem of a technique when studying Ayurvedic medicine and since blocked nasal passages and sinus issues can result in eye puffiness, is definitely worth a try.

Take a tiny glass bowl, fill with half teaspoon of **sea salt** and lukewarm water (which has been previously boiled). Holding right nostril closed with thumb, inhale the mixture through your left nostril until you feel its saltiness trickle down your throat. Repeat with the other nostril and have a good blow into a hankie. (You'll be surprised how much mucous comes out). The added bonus when done twice weekly is that it protects you from picking up colds – and I can honestly say I've been cold-free for years.

BEAUTY REMEDIES FOR BLACKHEADS, PIMPLES AND ACNE

*'Do things your future self
will thank you for.'*

If you suffer with pimples, acne, skin rashes or skin allergies, here are some ways to help cure them. There are no overnight cures since what needs to be corrected starts on the inside so it could take a month (or more) until you see results.

Let's start with something you know but might not be taking seriously enough, which is of course – diet. When our blood sugar levels are out of balance it causes hormonal fluctuation which in turn encourages acne. Therefore, if you've got pasta, white rice, white bread, white sugar, processed breakfast cereal, naughty potato chips or cake on your shopping list, cross them out and think whole grains, beans and vegetables.

Omega 3 has been shown to control the production of leukotriene B4, a molecule that is said to increase sebum. Excess sebum is one of the causes of skin eruptions. You could take an Omega 3 supplement every day or include walnuts, avocado, flaxseed oil and salmon in your diet since these are all rich in Omega 3 fatty acids which help to combat sebum.

Carrot Juice is packed with essential vitamins, minerals and antioxidants which can greatly improve dry skin conditions such as psoriasis.

Beetroot Juice is effective in reducing pigmentation, skin discoloration and blemishes.

If you don't have time to make your own juices, buy ready prepared cartons. For extra health/taste benefits, I add a good squeeze of lemon juice and a teaspoon of fresh grated ginger to mine.

Now think of skin outbreaks. They are hot. They rage. Take the rage out of them by wetting a face flannel, sprinkling with **witch hazel lotion**, protecting flannel in zip lock bag and leaving in deep freeze. Once a day, hold ice-cold flannel over face for 30 seconds and pop back in deep freeze for further use. (Rinse flannel out thoroughly every three days and sprinkle with fresh witch hazel).

Anise Star. The easiest way to make this acne facemask is to use a couple of drops of essential anise star oil, although you can also grind an anise star with a pestle and mortar if you have some in your cupboard.

Two drops **anise star** oil. 1 tbs **coconut oil.** 1 tsp **honey,** few drops of **lemon juice,** pinch of **Turmeric** powder. 2 drops **Lavender oil.**

If your coconut oil is solid, soften slightly by placing in dish over pan of boiling water then add all other ingredients and give it a good stir. Apply to face, leave on for 15 mins then rinse off with warm water.

Basil. A cup of basil tea every day will encourage your skin to become clearer since it purifies the blood and is a must for those with skin blemishes/acne due to its amazing anti-bacterial and anti-fungal properties. Just break off a few sprigs from a fresh basil plant, seep in boiling water for ten minutes, remove leaves and drink.

We can take basil a step further by transforming it into a healing face mask by whisking a handful of **basil leaves** in blender with 4 drops **lemon juice.** Beat with one egg white, add 2 drops Lavender oil then apply to skin for 15 minutes before rinsing off with warm water.

On a spiritual level, Basil is a herb which is said to protect us against negative energy attacks from those who show aggression or prove argumentative during the day. I often put a few drops of Basil oil in my palms and run lightly over my body after showering to protect my energy field when not feeling my warrior-like self.

Egg white can also be used for pimples. Beat an **egg white,** add 1 tbs finely grated **cucumber** and 2 drops **Lavender**

oil. Apply to face, leave for 20 minutes then rinse off with warm water.

Orange Peel. A great source of Vitamin C which combined with a little milk is another great mask to help cure blackheads and to nourish dry skin. Fruit peels, particularly orange or grapefruit help to clean skin by extracting dirt that gathers in the pores. Grate skin from half an orange (or grapefruit), add just enough milk to make a thin paste. Apply to face, leave for 5 mins and rinse off with warm water.

Parsley. Steep a handful of parsley in a cup of boiling water for 30 minutes. Strain and apply with a cotton wool pad to the face. Leave for 15 minutes. Wash off. Apply daily until pimples have disappeared.

Pureed (fresh) Apricots work as a fantastic natural home remedy for pimples and blackheads. Take two ripe apricots, cut them and remove the stone. Blend the fruit along with two tbs **honey** and 2 tbs **ground almonds** in food mixer. Apply to skin, leave on for 30 mins then rinse off with warm water.

CELEBRITY BEE STUNG LIPS

'And frankly my dears I don't give a damn if no-one but me gets me.'

You can watch me make this cinnamon, cayenne lip plumper on my YouTube channel. The title of video is as above.

This recipe contains potent herbs **Cinnamon** and **Cayenne** and **Peppermint** essential oil. These combined ingredients not only plump lips but nourish them so that they don't chap so easily.

And here's another benefit. The colours of cinnamon and cayenne give your lips a natural rosy glow so you don't need to apply lipstick. (I would add that cinnamon is said to be an aphrodisiac so I will not be held responsible for any shenanigans you might get up to when wearing this lip balm).

All you need are: 2 tablespoons **petroleum jelly** – in this case better than coconut oil since petroleum jelly acts as barrier to push other ingredients into lips. I sometimes warm petroleum jelly in plate over small saucepan of boiling water so that it's easier to work with but you can use straight from jar. 1 tsp **cinnamon** powder. Half tsp **cayenne** powder. 3 drops **peppermint** oil.

Initially the sting might feel too intense since this recipe is one which works best for my lips. If this proves the case, decrease the amount of cinnamon or replace with a tsp of ginger powder. Want bigger lips? Increase amount of cinnamon.

Mix thoroughly. Transfer to little pot and its ready for use sweet vixens.

CELLULITE/STRETCH MARK/SCAR SOLUTIONS

'There is no try. We do or do not.'

Who doesn't enjoy a good cup of coffee eh – but did you know that the caffeine in coffee provides antioxidants thus tightening the skin and reducing the appearance of cellulite when applied topically?

Caffeine stimulates skin cells and using it as a scrub gets rid of dead skin. Applied on a daily basis, it reduces the appearance of cellulite. This I can confirm since I've been scrubbing it into my thighs for the past month to prepare for a much looked forward to cruise.

My favourite caffeine cellulite fix is this:

Combine a tbs **coffee grounds** with two tbs **coconut oil** and a tsp **sea salt**. Once you've had a good scrub with your loofah, rinse off and follow with this generation old beauty secret from the Australian Aboriginal women.

Namely, it's **Yarrow Root**. It is used in face and body creams (normally found in health shops). Yarrow root contains anti-inflammatory compounds that not only heal most kinds of skin irritations but reduce the appearance of scars and stretch marks.

Essential oils are also a tremendous help when it comes to dealing with scars and stretchmarks. I particularly like **Neroli, Carrot seed and Frankincense**. You could use just one but as a team they're formidable and help to regenerate new skin as they fade old scars.

I bought a jar of Yarrow Root cream last year because I wanted to try it out on a scar on my leg (left behind by melanoma cancer op). For me, no cream without the addition of essential oils has true worth so I added 4 drops each of Neroli, Carrot Seed and Frankincense oil to give it extra healing power.

Was it my imagination that after three weeks the scar began to fade, or would that have happened anyway? I made a pot for further testing and gave it to a friend who had stretchmarks. She swore there was a difference.

I guess the point of my little story is that should you have stretchmarks, cellulite or scars, you might want to try my Yarrow Root cream recipe.

Since I was talking about Neroli oil a little earlier, I must talk more about its awesomeness. I'm not a stressful type but do suffer with occasional insomnia and that feeling of being down without knowing why. My remedy for this is to give myself a pamper bath with ten drops of Neroli oil. (I also use a squirt of Foamy Forest Fern Milk Bath Oil for which you can find recipe at back of this book in Xmas Gift Ideas). Neroli oil has sedative qualities which also lift mood so is brilliant for nervous, anxious types as well as for those who lack confidence. For hours after a Neroli bath, I can smell its deliciousness on my skin and feel its calming effect.

I put a few drops of Neroli oil on the inside of my wrists if I'm going to an important meeting. My meetings tend to go well so I'll carry on the same.

CHILDREN'S HEALTH RECOVERY CURES

'When you were little you promised yourself great things. Don't give up on yourself now.'

My daughter was used to seeing my face slathered in avocado as I chased her around the kitchen and begged her to try out a new beauty recipe. 'I'm not putting food on my face', she'd scream. I had similar problems when she was under the weather. I literally had to tie her to the bed to administer my natural health remedies. She called me cuckoo back then. Now she calls me *Cuckoo but Cool*, joins me in beauty pamper nights and cures herself with the remedies I once forced down her throat.

The recipes given hereunder cover a small cross section of the most common ailments children tend to suffer from, together with my suggestions on how to lessen using essential oils.

Asthma. When I think asthma, I think Rosemary, Pine, Benzoin, Thyme and Lavender oil. They're a perfect combination to ease asthma symptoms.

First, we need to make a massage oil – to rub into the child's chest. Let's make a 100ml bottle recipe. To a 100ml (glass) bottle, pour in almost 100ml of **sweet almond oil**, add 8 drops of **Benzoin** oil, 2 drops **Lavender** oil, 2 drops **Thyme** oil. Screw bottle top on, give it a good shake and your massage oil is ready for use.

Make sure any asthmatic child has a hot daily bath with 6 drops Benzoin, 3 drops Rosemary oil and 3 drops Thyme oil sprinkled into the bath water. Sprinkle a few drops of Rosemary oil on the child's pillow before he/she goes to sleep.

OK. This tip to ease asthma symptoms might not be easy to implement but should you happen to be somewhere that sells pine cones, buy a packet. Place them in a glass or wooden dish. Sprinkle cones with 4 drops each of Benzoin, Rosemary and Thyme oil. If you want to go that extra mile, buy a bottle of essential **Pine oil** and use that instead of 4 drops Rosemary oil.

Coughs. To a 100ml bottle of **sweet almond oil**, add 8 drops **Eucalyptus** oil, 3 drops **Pine** oil and 3 drops **Thyme** oil. Screw bottle top on, shake, and your massage oil is ready. Massage it into child's throat and chest until the cough symptoms ease.

Diarrhea. A Canadian research programme showed that 227 of 300 infants given **Carob Powder** in their formula milk, got relief from diarrhea. Carob has a high level of fibre which is just what we need to bind loose stools.

Dry Eczema. The best essential oil for dry eczema is **Geranium.** It has tremendous healing qualities for itchy, flaking skin and is often recommended for children's skin issues. This massage oil can be applied to affected areas as often as you wish.

Tip 8 drops of **Geranium** oil into 100ml bottle of **avocado oil**. Screw bottle top on. Shake. Your massage oil is ready for use.

Fear and Anxiety. Children imagine monsters, fret about exams, stress over their appearance and worry they don't fit in.

Homeopathic remedies are wonderful. However, they are not always enough to get into the child's psyche and do better partnered with essentials oils - for massage purposes, vaporized, to bathe in, smell or inhale. These awesome gems not only work on physical aspects of the face and body, they balance the brain and soothe the soul. (What a loving God we have to provide us with such help).

This recipe combines 5 essential oils, which between them work on stress, anxiety, irritability and fear.

Simply add 4 drops each of **Chamomile, Geranium, Lavender, Neroli and Thyme** oils to a 100ml bottle of carrier oil. Screw on top, shake and you're ready to use as suggested above.

Hiccups. I remember lots of hiccup tips from my childhood. Dad used to put a cold silver tablespoon down the back of my blouse to try and stop them. Mum would make me swallow a piece of crushed ice. Gran applied pressure to my eye balls then made me eat honey followed by a teaspoon of vinegar. Their remedies, based on shock tactics, worked more often that not so have a go the next time your child gets hiccups.

Travel Sickness. Before you're due to go on a journey, make this to take with. Tip 8 drops of **Peppermint oil** into a 100ml bottle of sweet almond oil. Screw top on. Massage this mixture into your child's tummy and behind his/her ears before you leave the house. Should the child start to feel sick, give them a peppermint oil scented handkerchief to sniff.

Tummy Ache. One of the best things for a tummy ache is a soft, soothing massage but we can improve on this by adding essential oils. Tip 3 drops of **Chamomile** and 3 drops **Rose** oil into 30ml bottle of **sweet almond** oil. To use, gently rub into child's tummy using circular motions.

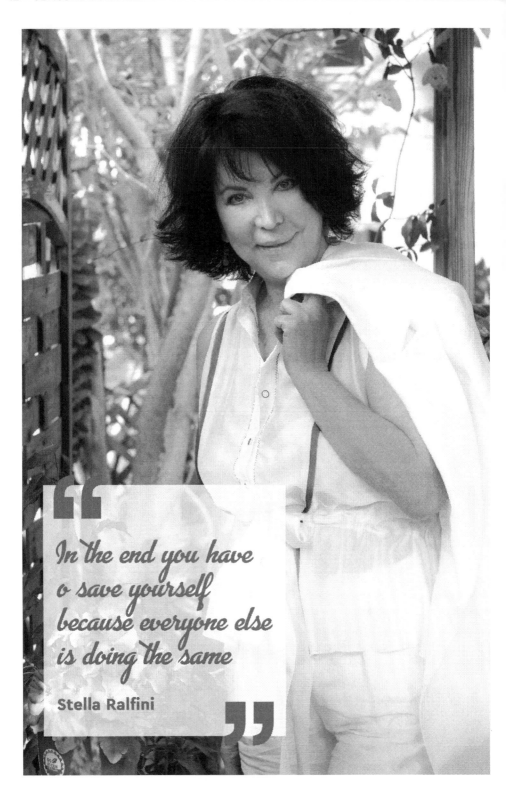

> In the end you have
> o save yourself
> because everyone else
> is doing the same
>
> **Stella Ralfini**

CHOCOLATE AND COFFEE DELIGHTS

*'If a girl wants to shake up the world
she should go ahead and do so.'*

I admit I'm a chocoholic who eats chocolate every day and often cover my face in it. No, not because I have a fetish. Because chocolate is a brilliant skin food.

Dark chocolate is superior since the antioxidants and compounds it contains, protects the skin from premature aging. It is also said to improve blood circulation, the result of which is radiant, glowing skin.

When giving myself a beauty session I normally combine two treatments. Exfoliator first then a face mask. I've found this double whammy approach to beauty pays off faster so it's worth doing two treatments when you can.

Chocolate/Coffee Exfoliating Scrub.

Heat 1 tbs **brown sugar** in 1 tbs **coconut oil** in dish over pan of boiling water. When the coconut oil melts, remove from heat and stir in 1 tsp finely ground **coffee beans** and 1 tsp **cocoa powder**. (This should be coarse enough but if you want a coarser texture, add 1 tsp oatmeal powder). Scrub your face and neck using gentle circular motions, rinse off and you're ready to apply your mask.

Chocolate with Green Tea Face Mask

Green tea is another great source of antioxidants and here by combining chocolate, we create a mighty skin regenerating mask.

Cover 2 **Green Tea bags** in just enough boiling water to seep through tea bags. Leave for five minutes to cool. Squeeze out water then split tea bags open and add leaves to 1 tbs **cocoa powder**, 1 tbs **honey** and 1 tbs plain Greek **yoghurt**. Apply the face pack to face and neck for twenty minutes then rinse with warm water.

Coffee Mask.

Face masks containing coffee are said to tighten loose skin and help with saggy jaw issues. I'm not convinced coffee has the power to lift saggy jaws (mine are starting to give into gravity), but it does seem to make the face look slimmer when used regularly and is worth a try for that reason.

Combine 1 tbs freshly brewed **coffee grinds** with 1 tsp **honey** and 1 tsp Greek **yoghurt** and mix well. Apply

mixture to skin concentrating on the jawline and neck.
Leave on for 30 mins then rinse off with warm water

DETOX DAY

'Sexy isn't about size but how you wear it.'

These one day detoxes not only ensures radiant, smooth skin, they promote good health and weight loss. Start to see your body as a temple, knowing every mouthful of food you put into your mouth is either adding or detracting from your health and beauty. On the subject of weight loss, until the mind is trained to become your servant (instead of your master), it might be better encouraging it in small bites? I personally don't like the word 'diet' which seems to cause the mind to rebel. If weight loss is part of your agenda, a once weekly detox day is a good place to start.

So, if you are ready Gods and Goddesses, let's begin to create your awesome temple.

Breakfasts consist of the following, which you can mix and swap around to suit.

Fresh fruit breakfast with grapes, grapefruit and orange. (Grapefruit is particularly beneficial since it stimulates kidneys, liver and entire glandular system). Muesli with chopped fresh apple. A pot of natural yoghurt. Small bowl of porridge.

Lunch ideas: cooked brown rice with mixture of any/all green vegetables. Large potato boiled with skin, cottage cheese and mixed leaf salad. Vegetable soup. Salad with whole sliced avocado.

Dinner ideas: Meals should be small since the metabolism slows down after 7pm. Stick to steamed or grilled meat or fish and green salads that contain any/all of following: fennel, chicory, carrot, beetroot. If you're vegetarian, add brown rice to your salad.

Drink at least six glasses of water, a cup of herbal tea after lunch and two glasses of either carrot or beetroot juice during your detox day. If you really can't go without coffee, limit to one cup per day.

EYES SPECIFIC BEAUTY/HEALTH RECIPES AND TIPS

'Be the woman you needed as a girl.'

Avocado (as you already know)**,** is high on my list of beloved fruits to fight wrinkles since it contains tons of elements that positively affect skin.

Give a quarter of **avocado a** good mash, apply under eyes, leave on for 20 minutes then rinse off with warm water. You will have even better results if avocado is mixed with 1 tsp **Aloe Vera** gel.

Here is another very simple recipe to help eliminate wrinkles. All you are going to do is mix half a tsp **ginger powder** into half a tsp **honey**. (Honey acts as an excellent moisturizer for the skin and the ginger helps improve blood flow to the area where applied). Gently massage the mixture into area below and around the eyes), leave on for 20 mins then rinse off with warm water.

Vitamin C has been found to increase collagen production, correct pigmentation problems and improve inflammatory skin conditions. However, according to studies at Tulane University, the most potent type of Vitamin C to stop wrinkles forming is L-ascorbic acid so you may wish to consider taking a course.

Coconut oil is very effective when it comes to helping remove dark circles from under the eyes. Massage a few drops under them on a daily basis to achieve faster results.

Milk can prove a saviour for exhausted eyes. In this recipe we are also going to use **baking soda** to tighten the skin. Simply blend 4 tbs of fresh whole milk and 2 tbs of baking soda. Blend well to achieve a smooth consistency. Place it in the refrigerator and apply the chilled milk mask around your eyes. Leave on for 20 minutes and rinse off with cold water.

Turmeric Powder and Pineapple Juice. This is an effective remedy for eye bags which again, is super simple to make.

Mix quarter tsp **turmeric powder** into 1 tbs **pineapple juice** and stir for 30 seconds. Apply with clean fingers to under eye area, leave on for 20 minutes then rinse off with warm water. Women I recommend this treatment to tell me its one of their favourites to deal with eye bags but as with every other recipe, nothing's going to change if you do any treatment once – so here I repeat what helps me to keep looking foxy tailed – *Repetition and dedication.*

Cottage Cheese. Yes, who would have thought that cottage cheese would be something I'd recommend that you use on your eyes eh but it does a great job of getting rid of eye puffiness. Put a small amount of cottage cheese on two cotton pads, place them over your closed eyelids, leave on for ten minutes then rinse eyes with warm water.

Yoghurt and Parsley. My gran swore by this recipe to get rid of dark circles so you may want to give it a go. (For your info, parsley contains beta-carotene, vitamin C, folic acid and minerals which even out skin tone and are said to prevent wrinkles).

All you need to do is finely crush a tsp of **parsley leaves** and mix well into a tbs plain **yoghurt**. Apply mixture around eyes, leave on for 10 minutes then rinse off with cool water.

Did you notice what I missed out in this batch of recipes? Essential oils. I feel you have reached the stage where you know enough to select one by yourself so go back over the essential oils used at the beginning of this book and choose 2 drops of whichever one feels right and add to the recipe you want to work with.

EGGS FOR SKIN EXCELLENCE

Since you're gonna dream, dream huge.'

As a child, there was nothing I liked better than a soft-boiled egg with buttered toast soldiers to dip in.

One day mum suggested I put egg white on my face to get rid of the pimples on my cheeks. The only reason I went along was that I didn't want to be a pimply teen and would have tried anything. My egg white masks must have helped since my skin cleared up, but why did mum give me egg white and keep the yolk for her?

This is the difference.

Egg White absorbs excess oil from the skin, while eking out impurities that cause acne, pimples and other skin disruptions.

Egg Yolk is mainly made up of water and fats which act as a water-binding agent to lock moisture into the skin, thereby nourishing and hydrating it in the process.

Egg White, Lime and Grapefruit Mask for Oily Skin

Add one **egg white**, juice of quarter **lime** (or lemon) to a bowl. Grate rind from half a **grapefruit** then add to mixture. Sprinkle 2 drops **Lavender oil** into mixture, beat thoroughly and apply to face and neck. Leave on for 20 minutes then rinse off with warm water.

Wrinkle Busting Egg Yolk Mask.

I love this mask since it can also be used to help remove wrinkles around the lips as well as around the eyes and is oh so simple to make.

Mix one tsp **honey** with one tsp **Argan oil**, into an **egg yolk** and whisk thoroughly. Apply around eyes and lips. Leave on for 30 mins then rinse off with warm water.

Face Plump Mask for all skin types.

Another brilliant face mask which uses the qualities of both egg white and egg yolk. The **turmeric/honey** combination act as a stimulant to plump the skin. By now you know the benefits of the essential oils we use.

.2 tbsp **Aloe Vera Gel**. 1 beaten **egg**. Quarter tsp **turmeric** powder. 1 tsp **honey**. 4 drops **Geranium**, **Rose** or **Frankincense** oil.

Mix the Aloe Vera gel, egg, turmeric, honey and essential oil of choice until you have a smooth consistency. Apply to the face and neck. Leave mask on for 30 minutes then rinse off with warm water.

Mint and Cucumber Revitalizing Egg White Face Mask

This is a great mask to use in the summer months when you've been exposed to the sun (and I don't mean sun bathing 'cause that's gonna age you faster than anything).

Apart from egg white, our main ingredients are mint and cucumber. Both **mint** and **cucumber** have a cooling effect on the skin whilst energizing and tightening it.

Mash quarter **cucumber** in a food processer then strain. Place cucumber solids in small saucepan with a teaspoon of **rose water** and simmer until warm. Stir in quarter cup of finely chopped fresh **mint leaves**. Simmer for another minute. Leave to cool. Add slightly whipped **egg white**. Look at essential oil category at the beginning of my book. Choose one that you feel is appropriate for your skin type and add 3 drops. Mix well then apply to face and neck. Leave for 20 minutes. Wash off with **cold** water.

Egg White Facial Hair Remover. I think it was first in Ecuador that I saw a woman use egg white to remove facial hair. I didn't try it due to the fact I had my facial hair zapped out with electrolysis in my twenties but she swore by her egg white trick.

All you need is a slightly whipped egg white and a piece of kitchen towel paper (the sort we use to wipe down surfaces).

Apply **egg white** to your face with a brush (make up or pastry), cut holes for your eyes and mouth in a piece of paper towel, press the paper towel to your face then coat with more egg white to make it stick. Once it is completely dry, quickly pull off towel and voila. No more fuzz.

ESSENTIAL OIL MUST HAVES

'Don't take love too seriously. It's as fickle as the next breath.'

Essential Oil Facial Serum and Skin Tightening Spritzer

Before you make any other recipes in this book, these two are musts. I have been using both daily for the past ten years and believe they could be the reason my skin's still so supple. However, I give my face such regular love, I can't be certain which treatments do the most anymore but there is proof this serum works since I also massage it into my hands which look strikingly young.

I created the tightening spritzer to compliment the facial serum. They've proved a good team, are suitable for all skin types and I guarantee that once you've used them for three months you will choose to use forever. One bit of advice. Use just a tiny amount of oil serum to begin with. Once your skin gets used to it and absorbs the oils you can try with more.

Essential Oil Facial Serum.

Who would have thought that such an effective treatment takes less than 30 seconds to make? All that you are going to do is transfer just under 30ml **Apricot Kernel** oil to an empty 30ml glass dropper bottle. Add 4 drops each of **Rose, Frankincense and Geranium** oil and half tsp **Evening Primrose** oil. Replace dropper top, gently shake and it's ready to use.

Essential Oil Skin Tonic Spritzer.

Another recipe you can make in the blink of an eye that tightens skin with regular use.

Pour just under 100ml of **Rose Water** into an empty glass spray bottle. Add 8 drops **Rose** oil, 6 drops **Frankincense** oil, 6 drops **Lavender** oil, 1 drop **Grapefruit** oil, 1 drop **Orange** oil. These won't disperse in the Rose Water unless we add either a tsp of **witch hazel** or **vodka** to break them down, so add a tsp of either to your mixture. Replace spray bottle top and give your skin tonic a good shake. Transfer to refrigerator and use from there morning and night on clean skin.

You can watch me make both recipes on my YouTube Channel.

GLYGOLIC ACID FRESH FRUIT FACE PEELS

'Don't take life too seriously. It's as fickle as the next breath.'

Glycolic acid face peels are a popular treatment in beauty salons these days but why spend money when we can make excellent peels at home? Glycolic acid is a natural derivative of sugar cane and a member of the alpha hydroxyl acid (AHA) tribe. Natural acids and enzymes are found in fruits. Combine these two heroes and we have a super exfoliating peel which also helps to close pores and brightens skin.

Dependent on ingredients used, we can make our peels mild or strong. My two recipes suit all skin types, other than ultra-sensitive.

Apple-Orange Glycolic Acid Peel

Few drops of **Rose Water**. 1 tsp white **sugar.** 1 tbs **honey.** 2 tbs baby **apple sauce.** 1 tsp **orange juice**. 1 tsp **grated orange peel.** 2 tbs **ground oatmeal.**

Combine rosewater with sugar, honey, apple sauce, orange juice/grated orange peel and oatmeal. Mix well with handle of wooden spatula.

Apply to face and neck with clean fingers (avoiding eyes), leave on for 15 minutes then dab face with warm water and gently scrub off. To take treatment a step further and tighten pores, run an ice cube over face and neck for 30 seconds.

Pineapple-Grapefruit Glycolic Acid Peel.

Take half cup **fresh cut pineapple**, (you can buy ready prepared tubs in supermarkets), Mix with 2 tsp **grapefruit juice** and **grated rind** from half a **grapefruit**.

Blend together in blender, add half tbs **honey** and mix together. If you want to add skin tightening effect while skin is gently peeling, mix in half a well beaten **egg white.** Apply mask to face and neck, leave on for 20 minutes then rinse off with warm water.

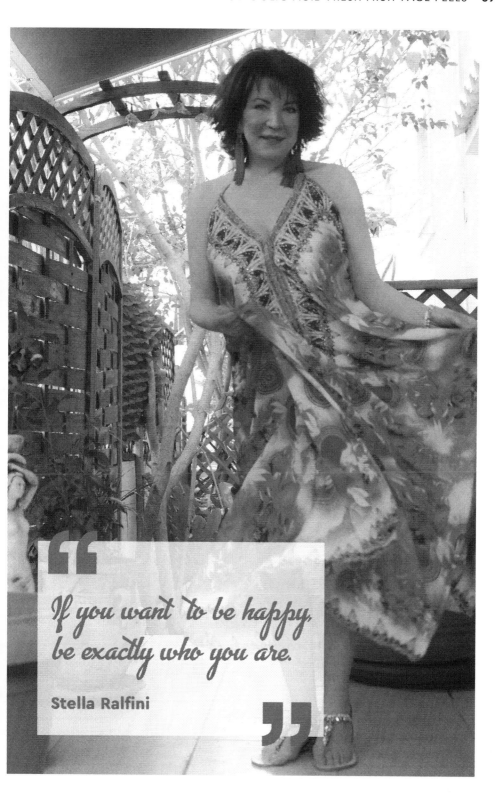

If you want to be happy, be exactly who you are.

Stella Ralfini

HAIR AND NAIL STRENGTHENING BEAUTY MUST KNOWS

'Don't take age too seriously.
Don't die before you're dead.'

When I posted a picture of my hand on Facebook, people asked how I keep mine so young looking so let's address that issue.

Exfoliate once a week with a teaspoon of **brown sugar** mixed into a tablespoon of **olive oil,** rub vigorously over back of hands then rinse off with warm water.

If you have dark spots, lessen them by exfoliating twice weekly with tablespoon of **lemon juice** mixed into heaped teaspoon of **white sugar** before rinsing off with warm water.

A daily hand massage works wonders. Mix a few drops of **Rose oil** with a blob of **coconut oil** and lightly massage into hands, fingers, nails and cuticles (If you have already made it, you can use a little of your **Essential Oil Facial Serum** on your hands like me).

Once a week must do for your hands is to coat them with thin layer of **petroleum jelly** before you go to bed. Put on a pair of white cotton gloves and leave them on overnight (buy gloves from any pharmacy).

Always apply SPF50 sunscreen before going out and apply hand cream when at home. The above is what I do and it seems to be working fine so far. Over to you beautiful all.

Brittle Breaking Nails

I gave my nails this treatment a few years back when for some reason they started to flake. This recipe strengthened them.

Combine 2 tsp **salt** with 1 tsp **wheat germ oil**, 2 tsp **castor oil**, 2 tsp **carrot seed oil**, 2 drops **Lavender** oil and mix well. Place in tight fitting jar to store. When you want to use, coat cotton pad with mixture and massage into nails and cuticles. Leave it on for 5 mins then wipe clean. For maximum results, you should give yourself this treatment three times a week for four weeks by which time your nails will feel like granite.

Grape and Sugar Nail Strengthener

For this beauty tip I must thank my (now deceased) aunt in Cyprus. That side of my family were all field workers. I will never forget my first visit. There was no electricity and the toilet, in an outside shed, was a hole in the ground that crawled with cockroaches. That proved a huge culture shock. However, I did learn about herbs, how to bake bread in a clay oven and gleaned beauty gems like this.

Cut five **grapes** in half, sprinkle with **granulated sugar** and leave for a few minutes to allow sugar to soak into the flesh of the grape.

Rub one grape half over thumb nail and into cuticle, then repeat with another sugared grape half on the other thumb nail. Give all your fingers the same treatment. Leave on for a few minutes then scrub off with a nail brush. My aunt had incredibly strong nails and followed the grape treatment with an **olive oil** hand massage to keep them soft.

Hair Strengthening Suggestions That Show Results.

Milk and honey are two ingredients that restore vitality to damaged hair. **Milk** is rich in minerals, vitamins, zinc, calcium which keep the hair healthy and shiny. It also contains whey protein and casein to help stop hair loss. **Honey** is a rich source of antioxidants which strengthens hair follicles and stops the hair from breaking.

Mix 1 tbs **honey** into half a cup of warm **milk** and stir until honey dissolves. Pour mixture over hair and massage into roots. Put on a shower cup so the milk stays there as opposed to running down your neck. Leave on for 20 minutes, rinse off with warm water and wash hair with your regular shampoo.

Dry, Brittle Hair seems to benefit with this hair mask which uses avocado, honey, olive oil and essential Lavender oil.

Whip a mashed avocado together with 1 tbs **honey,** 1 tsp **olive oil** and 6 drops of **Lavender** oil. Beat together until you have a smooth consistency.

Dip your fingers into the mixture and rub well into the ends of your hair. When that is done, rub what's left of your mixture into your scalp. Protect head with shower cup, leave on for 20 mins then rinse off and shampoo as normal.

Super Simple Egg Mask for Beautiful, Thick Hair.

I'm not going to start talking about eggs again because you've heard me rave enough, so let's just get on with this recipe for shining, silky locks.

Beat two eggs in a bowl. (If you have short hair you can use one egg). After thoroughly beating, rub the egg into your hair and cover with a shower cap. Leave the egg in for about 20 minutes then rinse off and shampoo as normal.

Coconut milk, olive oil and Rosemary oil. Here's a wonderful combination to soften and condition hair since both olive and Rosemary oil have antiseptic properties which work well on dry scalp conditions. Coconut milk is loaded with vitamins like niacin and folate that give hair such a healthy shine, people will look at yours and say *Wow*. If you fancy a bit of *Wow,* here's what to do:

Mix together quarter cup of **coconut milk**, (you can buy cartons of coconut milk in supermarkets) 1 tsp **olive oil** and 5 drops **Rosemary** oil.

Using a wide toothed comb, carefully comb mixture through hair, paying special attention to the ends.

Wrap head in a warm towel for 20 minutes then rinse off and shampoo as normal.

And talking of grapes which we were earlier when I shared my Greek Cypriot aunt's nail strengthening recipe, here's her recipe to strengthen hair.

Half cup plain Greek yogurt. Half cup crushed seedless green grapes. Give ingredients a good blend then massage mixture into hair and scalp. Protect head with shower cap, leave on for ten minutes, rinse off and shampoo hair as normal.

HANGOVER CURES

'Don't let them box you in while you're still alive. Coffins are for the dead.'

I don't drink as much as I used to. Not through choice but because it takes me three days to get over a hangover. One day was bad enough, but since I had no intention of giving up alcohol back then, (yes, I veered towards wild in my youth), I knew there was only one answer. To find a cure to make the symptoms less nauseas.

You already know that you should try to eat at least a piece of toast for breakfast, avoid anything with milk and drinks loads of water to flush toxins out of your body. What you might not be aware of is the role essential oils can play to ease hangovers.

My first suggestion is a **cold compress**. For this, simply wet a face flannel, wring it out and place in freezer for 15 mins to get really cold. When you take it out of the freezer, sprinkle with 2 drops of **Peppermint** oil and 2 drops of **Lavender** oil and press to forehead and temples. This will help with the headache side of things (you can reapply compress as often as you wish).

Drinking copious glasses of water throughout the day will help to detoxify the liver but another way is to add 1 drop of **Rose** oil and 1 drop **Ginger** oil to a teaspoon of carrier oil and massage it into the liver area (this is just below the right side of your ribs).

These two tips helped, so you may want to give them a try the next time alcohol wins the battle.

Once when I was in Japan and drank enough sake to sink a ship, a friend gave me an **umeboshi plum** before I went to bed. Umeboshi plums, which are pickled, salted and soaked in green tea, have long been used as a traditional hangover remedy. Miraculously, I didn't wake up with a splitting headache the next morning and was so impressed I brought a jar back. (A jar of umeboshi plums are good to have even if you're not suffering with a hangover since they ease body aches, boost liver function and aid digestion).

Should you live in Scotland, I hear Glaswegian butchers swear by 'Irn-Bru' sausage as a hangover cure. It's made by replacing water with whisky.

HERB INFUSION SKIN TONICS

'Many will pat you on the back when you do good. Beware when you do better.

I make lots of herb infused tonics for clients to address specific skin issues and sometimes lean on the wisdom of Hippocrates, (considered to be one of the most outstanding figures in the history of natural medicine), to fire my brain cells.

If you have fresh herbs to hand even better but dried herbs also do a fine job. In our first recipe we are using thyme and fennel. **Thyme** because it's an antiseptic which is wonderful for reducing redness, healing spots and shrinking pores, and **fennel** for its gentle healing cleansing properties. If you have sensitive skin, this skin tonic is for you.

Thyme and Fennel Sensitive Skin Tonic.

2 tsp ground **fennel seeds**. 1 tsp dried **Thyme** (or a couple of fresh sprigs). Juice of half a **grapefruit** together with 1 teaspoon **grated grapefruit peel**. 4 drops **Tea Tree** oil.

Mix thyme and fennel in a bowl and cover with half a cup of boiling water. Leave for five minutes, add grapefruit juice, grapefruit peel and 4 drops Tea Tree oil. Allow mixture to steep for thirty minutes, strain infusion, transfer to squirt top glass bottle and place in refrigerator for use.

Sage Skin Tonic with Patchouli oil for oily skin.

Sage is a natural inflammatory often found in anti-aging serums and is believed to decrease puffiness and redness. Patchouli oil takes the oiliness out of skin and works on acne and skin eruptions.

3 tbs **dried sage**. Half tsp **apple cider vinegar**. 5 drops **Patchouli** oil. Throw sage into mug. Pour half cup of boiling water over 3 tbs dried sage. Leave to cool slightly and add one teaspoon apple cider vinegar. When completely cool, strain infusion and add Patchouli oil. Transfer to glass squirt top bottle, give mix a good shake and refrigerate for use.

Basil Skin Tonic with Frankincense oil

What can I say about Basil? I use it in tea, lotions, potions, salads, pasta dishes and wherever else I can. Here's a basil skin tonic recipe for normal, combination or troubled skin.

Crush handful fresh **basil leaves**, pour mug of boiling water over them and leave to completely cool. When cool, strain and add 5 drops **Frankincense** oil. Transfer into squirt top bottle, give mixture a good shake and transfer to refrigerator for use.

ICE BABY ICE – NATURAL INSTANT FACE LIFT

'Keep them alive. Dreams don't have an expiration date.'

You are probably aware that there are beauty treatments on the market that use the 'freeze' method to lift skin. I say why waste money when we have ice cubes in our freezers that do the job for free?

I can no longer remember where I picked up this tip but whenever I want to give my skin a tightened effect, I use ice.

My simplest tip regarding ice, is to run an ice cube around eyes, over face and neck for thirty seconds every morning before applying your daily face cream. As you'll see it brings an instant glow and makes skin fresher looking.

One day when I was running an ice cube over my face and ice dripped over my fingers I thought, 'Hold on, I can improve on this.' I saw how, tried it out then called friends to get them to have a go. The verdict was favourable as cries of 'I look like I've had a face lift,' shrieked back at me down the 'phone.

Before you give yourself an ice treatment, try this mini facial massage. It will increase results of the ice treatment since the ice will help to drive the oils into your skin.

Pour a tsp of **Argan oil** and 4 drops of **Frankincense oil** into a small glass bowl. Mix them together with a finger. Dip the fingers of both hands into the mixture so that they are coated in oil. Dab the oil over throat, face and around eyes until you use up the mixture in your bowl.

Bring your hands to your throat and gently flick skin under throat towards the chin with *fanned* fingers. Practice until it comes naturally. When you reach your chin line, pinch skin between your fingers and work towards your ears. Pinch your cheeks, working outwards towards your temples. When you arrive at your eyes, place *closed* fingers facing each other in the middle of your forehead. Using a firm touch, slowly stretch the skin on your forehead outwards towards your temples. Allow your fingers to move down to your cheek bones then forget about working towards the temples. This time, using a gentler touch, run your fingers inwards along your cheek bone towards your nose several times then rest your fingers on the inside of your nose. Using your finger pads, imagine you are erasing any fine lines between your eyebrows as you keep nudging skin upwards and outwards towards your forehead.

Well done you. That was an excellent first try. You are ready for the final stage.

Take 3 or 4 **ice cubes**, wrap them in a cloth napkin, twist the ends, place ice parcel on plate, wait for 30 seconds to allow coldness of ice to seep into napkin and your ice cube tool is ready for use.

Run your ice cube tool over your neck and face three times. Use upward, outward strokes other than under the eyes. Look in the mirror. Uh-hu…I said you'd love the result Ice Queens.

OATMEAL. A SECRET BEAUTY WEAPON OF PAST GENERATIONS

'I needed my past and my mistakes to get me where I am now.'

As a child I had oatmeal for breakfast quite a lot. As an adult, I learned that oatmeal could be used to effectively treat skin rashes, inflammation, eczema and wrinkles. These days I'm back to eating it regularly since it helps to keep my cholesterol down.

All the ancient skin pros knew about oatmeal as a beauty ingredient and what a gem it is. Oatmeal contains chemicals known as saponins. Saponins have excellent cleansing properties which inhibit the spread of bacteria and help to shrink pores while moisturizing and softening skin.

I could write a book on oatmeal uses but shall curb my enthusiasm so we don't overdose and will stick to four that focus on wrinkles. Wrinkles seem to be a woman's number one concern, on which note I offer this advice. Do not start on Botox too young. All it does is stretch the muscles – which sag back when the Botox wears off. Each time it wears off you'll become more wrinkle aware and imagine yours getting deeper – and they might be because when the muscles are stretched, it inhibits the production of natural collagen. There are better beauty treatments on the market than Botox.

If you would like to read about what they are and what I do three times a year to help fight gravity's pull, check out my article 'Where to Find Natural Beauty Makeovers at a Fraction of The Price.' You will find it under the Health and Beauty tab on my website (stellaralfini.co.uk)

Oatmeal Face Mask for Dry, Flaky Skin

This recipe calls for cooked, still slightly warm oatmeal so that it penetrates the pores, and in the process exfoliates. Let's take a look at what we need.

Oatmeal. Raw Honey. Egg Yolk. Argan oil. Rose oil.

Mix half a cup cooked, warm **oatmeal** into 1 tbs raw **honey**, 1 **egg yolk**, 1 tbs **Argan oil** and 4 drops **Rose oil**. Blend until you have a paste like a cake mix, apply to face and neck for 30 mins then rinse off with warm water.

Wrinkle Busting Oatmeal Face Mask

I created this mask for older women but that doesn't mean younger folk wouldn't benefit from a treatment. It needs just four ingredients, which are:

Oatmeal, 1 egg, 1 tbs apple sauce, 4 drops Frankincense oil

Mix half cup *cooled,* cooked **oatmeal** into 1 **egg**, 1 tbs **apple sauce** and 4 drops **Frankincense** oil. Blend until you have the consistency of a cake mix, apply to face and neck for 30 mins then rinse off with warm water.

Oatmeal and Celery Hydrating Mask

I love **celery.** It's one of my favourite vegetables and as with every other vegetable, I'm in awe of its powers to heal and beautify. Due to the fact that celery is packed with enzymes, antioxidants, essential minerals, vitamins A, K and magnesium, it has the ability to lower tumor activity, lower blood pressure, treat arthritis, age related vision loss and more. Celery is also a master player in the beauty field and known for restoring hydration to the skin. Here's a recipe to ease those wrinkles out.

2 tbs powdered uncooked oatmeal, 2 tbs celery juice, 3 drops Lavender oil.

Juice a couple of sticks of celery. Extract 2 tbs celery juice, mix into powdered uncooked oatmeal and add Lavender oil. Blend until you have a paste and apply to face and neck. Leave on for 20 min then wet your hands and gently scrub the mask away in circular motions. Rinse off with warm water. Pat skin dry and run ice cube over face and neck for 30 seconds.

Sassy Oatmeal/ Ginger Mask
(enough for three treatments)

The ingredient I adore in this recipe is the **fresh ginger**. In Ayurvedic medicine, ginger is hailed as a solution for dark spots, scars and lightening skin tone. I take a tsp of grated fresh ginger, mixed into a tsp of honey every day to boost my immune system and clear my lungs (sorry to disappoint some but I still smoke 5-7 roll ups a day). I use fresh ginger in the fruit and vegetable juices I drink and use it in tons of beauty recipes. Here's a mask to use three times within nine days to give your skin added oomph.

All you need is: 4 tsp powdered **oatmeal**. Half a cup of melted **coconut oil**. Good half tsp grated fresh **ginger**. 2 tsp **Evening Primrose oil**. 2 drops **Rose** oil. 2 drops **Patchouli** oil. 2 drops **Frankincense** oil

Mix together all the ingredients until you have a smooth consistency. Transfer to small glass screw top jar. When coconut oil hardens, keep refrigerated so that coconut oil stays solidified.

Using one third of mix, apply to face, neck and chest. Leave on for 30 mins. Before rinsing off, give your skin a rub to remove dead skin.

OVERNIGHT TRANSFORMATION WRINKLE SERUM

'Push yourself. No-one else is going to do it for you.'

What I love about this serum is that we leave it on overnight to burrow away at wrinkles. I used in four nights in a row and saw a noticeable difference. By using beeswax in this recipe, we form a protective shield on the skin which when mixed with the other ingredients, pushes them into it and creates a sealed wall around them. You can't see the wall. It's as thin as gossamer and works much in the way of petroleum jelly – without the gunky feel. I've experimented with this recipe quite a bit and like the consistency of this one. Having tried it, you might want something thicker. If so, slightly increase the amount of beeswax.

All you need are: 3 tsp **Jojoba oil**. 3 tsp **Apricot Kernel oil**. 1 tsp **Beeswax**. 3 tsp **Rosewater**, Eighth tsp **baking soda**. 5

drops **Frankincense** or 3 drops Frankincense and 2 drops **Geranium oil.**

Place beeswax in dish over a pan of boiling water. When it melts, add the Jojoba and Apricot Kernel oils. Warm Rosewater in plate over pan of boiling water. Add baking soda to rose water and beat well. Add that to beeswax mixture. Whip until its smooth and fluffy then add your essential oils. Transfer to small pot and leave to harden. Transfer to refrigerator and use from there.

Imagine the nourishment your skin gets with an overnight pamper? Make a point to give yourself this treatment on a regular basis.

PINEAPPLE, AGE DEFYING FACIAL TREATMENT PACKAGE

'If you don't like your life story write a new one.'

By chance, when I created this anti-aging pineapple treatment package, I discovered what proved (for me) a beauty **biggie**.

In the recipes below you will find out what that biggie is, but since they say the best should be left for last, let's not rush things. I would like you to try out the first two suggested beauty treatments before going in for the final kill. That way your eyes will see the difference – and trust me, you'll be thrilled.

While a little messy, recipes are easy and results can prove phenomenal. For the first part of your pineapple beauty package, you need four ingredients.

A Fresh Pineapple. Honey.
Coconut Milk. Rose Water.

Before we get started on making our recipes though, let's recap on the benefits of the ingredients.

Pineapple: Packed with vitamin C and powerful antioxidants that not only stimulate skin but the immune system, plus pineapple is excellent for keeping eyes healthy and bones strong.

Honey: Packed with antioxidants to nourish/soothe skin and give it a beautiful glow.

Coconut milk: Rich in fibre, VIT C,E,B1,B3,B5, B6, iron, selenium, calcium, magnesium and phosphorous so not only great for skin but for strengthening hair and nails.

Rose Water: The antioxidants in rose water protect skin cells. Since it is anti-inflammatory, it can be used to soothe irritations caused by eczema and rosacea.

Assuming you have your ingredients to hand as well as your essential oils, let's get cracking.

Fresh Pineapple Exfoliator

Cut the fresh pineapple at the top (stalk end) so that you have a half an inch slice of pineapple with stalk still attached. This has now become an excellent exfoliating tool. All you're going to do (holding stalk), is to gently rub pineapple flesh over your face and neck. Use small circular motions and keep rubbing into skin for at least a minute. Leave on (you will start to feel it tingle) and make your next recipe.

Pineapple Pore Minimizing Super Nourishing Mask

1 tbs fresh blended **pineapple.** 1 tbs **Rose Water**, 1-2 tbs **honey**. Few drops **Frankincense, Rose or Lavender** essential oil. (I usually add a full tsp of regular yoghurt to this recipe so if you've got any in the fridge, go ahead and do the same).

This recipe is quite messy so you may wish to use a makeup or pastry brush to apply. Keep applying to face and neck until honey sticks to your skin then forget about it for 20 minutes. Rinse off with warm water - and wow you foxy minx, what glowing skin you have.

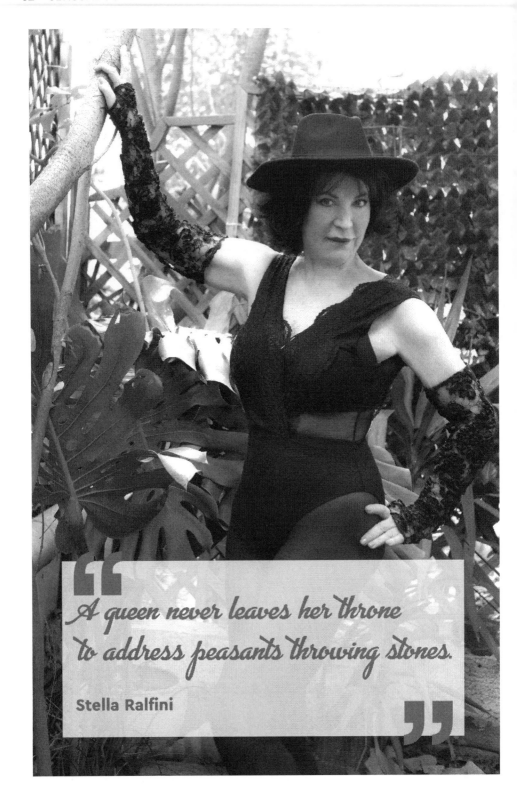

A queen never leaves her throne
to address peasants throwing stones.

Stella Ralfini

PINEAPPLE AGE DEFYING FACE LOTION

*'They said act your age.
I said I don't have one.'*

I told you earlier that in the process of working on my pineapple beauty package, I found a formula that makes skin look visibly tighter. Sure, it doesn't last. We're not talking plastic surgery. However, it's something that if you do regularly, will encourage your skin not to slack.

This recipe is crazily simple for the results. The four ingredients gel into a powerful team of face lift workers like few I've come across. Why these four ingredients fuse so well I'm not sure but they're the best combination I've tried so far.

All you are going to do is blend a quarter cup of fresh **pineapple juice** with 1 tbs **coconut milk** until completely smooth. Add 3 drops essential oil. **Lavender** for problematic/blemished skin. **Geranium** for all other skin types. Add half tsp **baking soda** and whip into mixture. Pour into a little glass dish. (You will have enough for **three** treatments which you should do three days in a row).

Dab clean fingers into pineapple mix and apply to face and neck in small circular movements. Leave to dry slightly and repeat this procedure twice more. Leave on for 20 mins, rinse off with warm water then dab face with rose water to tone. (As the third coat of pineapple liquid mixture starts to dry, you'll feel a slight itch, followed by a stronger tingle and will feel your skin begin to tighten).

The following day/evening, when you repeat what you did first time around, the enzymes in the pineapple will have further fused into the other ingredients to add extra zest to your mixture.

After my third night, I was so chuffed with the results, I patted myself on the back.

Give yourself the *complete* pineapple package beauty treatment once a month to keep results going.

POTATO

*'To get respect you first have
to respect yourself.'*

Yes, that potato in your kitchen is a killer beauty ingredient and this anti-aging mask couldn't be easier to make.

Potatoes have a high content of vitamins B and C, contain the mineral selenium and a variety of phytonutrients– important antioxidant enzymes when it comes to skin care. A once a week potato mask will help to reduce wrinkles, and due to its starch content will draw out dark circles and improve skin tone all round.

All you are going to do is grate a small **potato,** mix with 1 tbs plain **yoghurt,** 1 tsp of either **almond/coconut oil**, 1 tsp **honey,** 2 drops **Frankincense oil** and give it a good stir.

Apply around eyes to face and neck and leave on for 20 mins before rinsing off with warm water and I guarantee your skin will feel and look better

Potato is *the* vegetable to get rid of dark circles around the eyes. Whichever face mask I make, I often go that step further and cut a thin slice of potato in two pieces to place under my eyes while my face mask does its work. Normally I place the two thin slices of potato in a small bowl of cold water and leave in freezer for ten minutes before using so that the potato is really cold when I apply. This adds to the tightening effect and gives you two treatments in one.

Potato is also excellent for treating **freckles.** I personally love women with freckles but know that many don't so here's a freckle aid if you have them and wish to minimize.

Take 2 tbs horseradish, 1 tbs potato juice, (grate a small potato, place in cloth napkin and squeeze out the 1 tbs of potato juice you need). Add your two ingredients to a cup of **Sour milk** (you can buy Sour milk at supermarkets, you're not waiting for your milk to curdle lol). Allow to stand overnight. Add 4 drops **carrot seed oil.** (Carrot seed essential oil is super hero when it comes to dealing with hyperpigmentation and is super rich in beta carotene. The oil itself is extracted from carrot seeds and takes around 3000 carrot seeds to get one teaspoon of oil) Give your mix a final blend and apply to face with clean fingers. Leave on for 30 mins, rinse off with warm water and repeat treatment twice a week. Please remember to avoid strong sunlight and never leave home without sunscreen on your face.

STRAWBERRY AND RASPBERRY BEAUTY YUMS

'The wise don't expect life to be all sunshine. They weather storms with equal faith.'

Strawberry Cream Delight Anti-Aging face mask. During summer months, there is nothing more I enjoy than a delicious bowl of strawberries (ideally with a glass of champagne), but strawberries also have loads to offer when it comes to skin care.

Strawberries are not only rich in vitamin C, being acidic in nature they are excellent for removing excess sebum on skin as well as helping to lighten blemishes, so here's a mask for those with oily and/or discoloured skin that works well.

All you need is: Quarter cup mashed ripe fresh **strawberries.** 1 tbsp **single cream** (from a carton). 1 tbs **corn starch.** 4 drops **carrot seed oil.**

Give the ingredients a good blend then spread over face and neck. Leave on for 20 mins and rinse off with warm water. To make this treatment even more effective, when you take the mask off, give your face a massage with a few drops of carrot seed oil mixed into your carrier oil of choice. Voila, freckle face. Keep it up.

Note: You can also use leftover strawberries to whiten your teeth. Rub fleshy part of ripe strawberry all over them. Leave on for a minute, rinse off then brush teeth as normal.

Mixed Berry Face mask. I usually keep a packet of frozen berries in my freezer to use in exfoliating face masks throughout the year. This one's great for dealing with skin blemishes.

All you need to do is a quarter cup of frozen **mixed berries**, a quarter cup of **rolled oats**, and 1 tsp of **honey**.

Blend the ingredients together in an electric blender or food processor until you have a smooth paste. Sprinkle in 4 drops carrot seed oil, give mix a little whiz then spread the paste over your face and neck. Rinse off with warm water after 20 minutes and you'll see how much better your skin looks.

SENSUAL SORCERY IN THE BOUDOIR

'Make love your mantra. Make peace not war.'

Don Juan, who as you know was reported to be a veritable stallion in the boudoir and said to be at it day and night until he died, apparently drank this love potion an hour before sex to give him stamina. You need a glass of freshly squeezed **tomato juice.** Half a teaspoon of crushed **basil leaves**, 7 drops of **Chinese Ginseng** (liquid or squeezed from a capsule), a sprinkle of **cinnamon** and a pinch of **black pepper**.

For women with low libido, it was believed by ancient sexologists that a little powdered **clary sage** stirred into her glass of wine aroused sexual passion.

Cleopatra's Passion. This combination of fruits and herbs is a potent aphrodisiac which is also said to increase sexual appetite. It should be drunk an hour or so before love play begins.

Blend half a cup of **watermelon** (no seeds) with half a cup of **banana** and a cup of **papaya juice** (use tinned if fresh isn't available). Add half a teaspoon of powdered **cloves,** a good pinch of **nutmeg, saffron** and **cinnamon** and blend for ten seconds.

Ancient Sex stimulant. Here's a great tonic to build energy when his libido is low. Get him to drink it twice daily for three days and he won't know what hit him! Boil 6 chopped celery stalks with their leaves in 6 cups of water for five minutes. Let it steep for 15 minutes then remove celery. Add **black pepper, cinnamon, nutmeg** and a level tablespoon of honey to the liquid, (makes 6 cups).

Cupid's Douche. If you want to be sure your vagina smells (and tastes) like a flower garden, this once monthly douche is a must. Boil a quarter cup of **rose petals** in half a litre of water for one minute and remove the petals. Add half a teaspoon of good quality **apple cider vinegar** and half teaspoon of pure **honey.** Leave to cool, fill your douche bag and use as normal.

Korean Ginseng. Stimulates blood flow shortly before sex thereby helping male to maintain an erection. It is also said to increase testosterone levels.

Horny Goat Weed. This herb is found in Asia and the Mediterranean and is believed to help improve erectile function, increase libido and combat fatigue.

Shatavari. This herb, which is derived from a species of the asparagus plant, helps battle dryness, enhances fertility and nourishes the female reproductive organs.

Yohimbe. Bark stripped from a tree in West Africa. Said to stimulate circulation where you want it within an hour.

Tongkat Ali. A tree native to the jungles of Malaysia, Thailand and Indonesia, the root has long been used as an aphrodisiac.

Maca Root. This has been *the* herb for women living in the Andes for centuries. Maca's high iodine content supports a woman's hormone balance and its high zinc levels, (an essential mineral for sex hormones), does more than fan the flames of desire. Women who took Maca root in one study reported improved sexual experiences and satisfaction. You might want to put Maca on your shopping list!

(The above is an extract from my book *Three Faces of Sex*)

SPA BEAUTY/HEALTH DAY IN THE COMFORT OF OUR HOME

'If we want to win, we have to toughen up.'

You know what our problem is? We give ourselves so many responsibilities, we lose ourselves under the rubble. We spend our lives chasing trains, buses, careers and children. We don't stop to give ourselves the love we give others. We don't prioritize our wellbeing, our wants, or take time to indulge the soul. Self-love is not selfish. We need to love ourselves to find contentment. We'll do for others but *know* when to stop. There are many wolves out there. People who will eat us whole if we let them. I have boundaries. I take myself away from the world and prioritise *me* with an occasional beauty spa pamper at home. I play meditative music or House (depending on my mood) and light perfumed candles.

Are *you* ready to give yourself a spa treatment for the God or Goddess you are?

Here is what you need:

Loofah glove. Roll of **cling film** (to wrap around body) Small glass bowl filled with **sea salt.** Bottle of **Sweet Almond oil. Geranium and Rose oils**.

Ideally, you'll have already made a pot of my **Overnight Transformation Wrinkle Serum** to use?

Pre-prepare your avocado body/face mask and the Egg white and Rose essential oil nourishing face mask.

Avocado Body Mask
1 ripe **avocado.** 1 tbs **sea salt.** Eighth cup **honey. Grated rind** of 1 fresh **grapefruit.** Eighth cup **coconut oil**

Mix ingredients together in a bowl until you have a smooth consistency and you're done.

Egg White and Rose Oil Nourishing Face Mask
Beat **egg white** with half teaspoon **orange juice** and 3 drops of **Rose oil** until egg white is fairly stiff.

You are ready to set off for bathroom with your pre-prepped beauty goodies.

Once there, shower well, apply sea salt to wet body and scrub with loofah brush to remove dead skin.

Dry your skin then smear your legs, arms and chest with the avocado body mask. Take your roll of cling film and wrap around legs, arms and chest. This will stop it dripping and warm the body mask to help it penetrate your skin.

While your body mask is working its magic, apply egg white/rose oil mask to your face and neck. Leave both masks on for 20 mins then rinse off in the shower.

Pat skin dry and gently massage your body and face with quarter cup of sweet almond oil to which you've added 2 drops **Geranium** essential oil.

Hmm, think you can already see and feel a difference but it's time to add the final touch. Apply a thin layer of Overnight Transformation Wrinkle serum around your eyes, on face and neck, forget about it and leave on overnight.

Tomorrow when you wake up and feel how smooth your skin is, you will feel like a Goddess.

TAMARIND – ONE OF THE BEST KEPT BEAUTY SECRETS

'Bring it into reality by seeing it in technicolour.'

Tamarind not only tastes delicious in food recipes. Since it's packed with nutrients and vitamins, it's a *super-charged* fruit for glowing, clear, healthy skin.

Apart from magnesium, potassium, iron and phosphorous this amazing fruit contains niacin, vitamin C, calcium and copper. These tend to be used in expensive beauty products since they combat free radicals which are one cause of premature aging. Tamarind is also a wonderful source of alpha hydroxy acids (AHA), which eliminate impurities that lie deep within the skin so is excellent for use in exfoliating masks.

Tamarind can be bought in blocks, but it's a lengthy process to cut off a piece, soak for hours etc. I buy ready prepared Tamarind concentrated paste in jars which works just as well.

Here's an easy Tamarind exfoliating mask together with a Tamarind anti-aging mask that can be whipped up in no time.

Tamarind Exfoliating Mask

1 tsp concentrated **Tamarind paste**. 1 tsp **salt**. 1 tbs plain **yoghurt**, 3 drops **Lemon oil**.

Mix all ingredients until you have a smooth consistency, apply to face and neck, gently massage into skin for 3 mins to eliminate dead skin and rinse off with warm water. This mask really helps to close open pores so if this is one of your issues, repeat mask twice a week and you will see a noticeable difference.

Tamarind Anti-Aging Face Mask

The reason that expensive anti-aging products are such a hit is that everyone wants skin that doesn't show age and think the more they spend, the better the result. Here's an example of a homemade equivalent which is worth its weight in gold.

1 tbs concentrated **tamarind** paste. 1 tbs ground *****semolina flour**. 1 tsp **honey**. 4 drops **Frankincense oil**.

*Semolina flour is much healthier than all purpose flour, so you may wish to replace for your baking needs in the future.

Mix all the ingredients to form a smooth paste. Apply to face and neck, leave on for 30 mins then rinse off with warm water.

Tomatoes

Let me praise tomatoes for a moment before I move onto the beauty recipes. The juice of tomatoes contains a high percentage of nutrients that are beneficial for the skin. These include vitamin A, vitamin C, proteins and Lycopene. Lycopene is basically a carotenoid, which counteracts the damage of free radicals in the body. The abundance of Vitamin A and C, combats excess oils in the sebaceous gland so that we are not as prone to pimple outbreaks. Definitely a juice to consider drinking on a regular basis to promote health and clear skin.

Due to the vitamins, nutrients and carotenoid contained in tomato, it does a brilliant job of healing and nourishing skin. All you have to do is cut a ripe tomato in half and rub the fleshy part over your face and neck. Leave the juice on for 15 mins and rinse off with cold water.

Should you suffer with itching, redness or any form of skin irritation, the acidic qualities found in tomatoes help to regulate the skin PH level so here's a mask for that.

1 tbs of tomato juice mixed into three tbs of plain yoghurt.

Blend ingredients well then place in freezer for half an hour so that mixture hardens slightly. Apply to face and neck for 15 mins before rinsing off with ice cold water.

TWENTYFOUR HOUR BEAUTY MAKE OVER

'Never leave home without your Goddess charms. They're a woman's greatest weapon.'

Now, ladies, you know what I'm talking about. Some days you look in the mirror and think, 'Hell, is that *me*?' Maybe your look of saggy tiredness came about due to a passionate weekend of lovemaking. (those were the days lol). Maybe you know you weren't drinking enough water, overindulging or just being lazy with your beauty routine.

When I returned to Athens after six weeks nonstop travelling, my face looked exhausted and left me in no doubt it was time for an emergency measure beauty day.

Here's what it entails with health and beauty outline.

What to avoid: Coffee, meat, fish, processed foods, junk food – and whatever naughty treat normally tempts you.

What to include: Glass of warm water with half teaspoon fresh grated ginger and 3 slices of lemon when you wake up. One ounce of Pineapple juice mixed with one ounce of Papaya juice to drink immediately after lunch and dinner. (Papaya fruit contains the enzyme papain and pineapple contains the enzyme bromelain. Both enzymes aid the digestive system and combat stomach acid).

Breakfast: A homemade smoothie made with **almond, cashew or coconut milk**, half ripe **banana** and 1 fresh **kiwi** for breakfast. (Keep Kiwi skin and other half of banana for use in beauty treatments coming up).

Lunch: Salad or cooked vegetable dish with brown rice.
Snack: Small handful unsalted mixed nuts.
Supper. Tub of plain yoghurt

With that taken care of, let's move onto the face and the beauty treatments for your first beauty session of the day.

Exfoliator: Kiwi. Easy. Love. Remember you kept that kiwi skin when you had your smoothie this morning? You are about to use it to exfoliate. Give your face and neck a good rub with the fleshy part of kiwi skin. Leave it on for 10 mins and rinse off. (Kiwi is packed with Vitamin C to nourish and lighten skin, and enzymes to encourage new skin growth).

Tightening Egg White Mask. Crack an egg, separate the white from the yolk. (Keep yolk for evening beauty treatment). Whip egg white into a froth. Add 4 drops **Geranium** oil for older or combination skin or 4 drops **Lavender** oil for problematic skin.

Apply to face and neck with clean fingers or make up/ pastry brush. Leave on for 10 mins then rinse off with warm water.

Ice Treatment. Run an ice cube over your face and neck for 30 secs.

EVENING BEAUTY SESSION

Hydrating Nourishing Mask

This gives an instant glow effect.

1 egg yolk. 1 tsp olive or sweet almond oil, quarter ripe banana, 4 drops Rose or Lavender essential oil.

Mash banana with the back of a fork then slowly mix in egg yolk and oils until you have a smooth consistency. Apply to face, neck and eye area. Leave on for 25 minutes, rinse off with warm water. Cub ice cube over face and neck and apply night cream as normal.

You're ready for bed. It's time for another glass of almond, cashew or coconut milk to go on boosting your immune system while you dream of your next passionate weekend of lovemaking.

URINE THERAPY TO TREAT ACNE, ECZEMA, PSORIASIS AND WOUNDS

*'We are not what happened to us.
We are what we choose to become.'*

For me, Urine therapy is the winner cure for acne, eczema, psoriasis, pimples, wounds and scars. I've been singing its praises for years but it takes a certain mindset to accept.

Unbeknown to some of you, Urea (a chemical compound found in urine) is used as an ingredient in beauty products as well as topical creams (to deal with skin outbreaks). However, before I continue with how to apply, let's talk facts.

Urine is approximately 93% water. The other 7% is rich in with nutrients such as iron, magnesium, calcium and zinc and far from being toxic, urine is filtered twice before it leaves the body. Once by the liver and again by the kidneys. Toxic matter leaves the body via the faeces. Urine is completely sterile. Women of my mother's generation wiped babies down with their wet nappies as a cure for baby eczema. Urine is acclaimed in Ayurvedic and Chinese medicine and was favoured by the Aztecs to heal wounds - meaning I'm telling you nothing new since it has been around for centuries. (As opposed to what you might think, fresh urine does not smell when applied to your own body since it matches your DNA).

My introduction to urine therapy came in my thirties when I was studying Ayurvedic medicine in India. Distraught that my face was covered in weeping pimples, the doctor I was working under, said. 'Take a plastic cup, catch the middle flow of your urine in it then dab it on your face with a cotton pad twice a day for a week.'

Never a squeamish type, I followed his instructions and low and behold a week later my rash disappeared. In the 35 years I've been a beauty/health advisor, I've recommended it to clients who had skin issues. Each one was cured and are now urine therapy converts.

For those still in doubt, look at the bigger picture. Whatever supreme energy force created us, call it God or whatever you will, provided us with everything we need to naturally heal ourselves. Therefore, if you have a skin issue, open your mind to urine therapy.

XMAS COMES BEARING GIFTS

'Above all, don't lose hope.'

Ferny Forest Bath Oil.

Everyone who gets one of my bath oils for Xmas loves them. I love them because they are *so* easy to make. Just buy a 1000ml bottle of ready prepared foam bath gel and five 200 ml plastic bottles and you're ready to make five gifts.

For the Ferny Forest Bath Oil, pour just under 200ml of the bath gel into a bowl. Place half a tsp of dried thyme and rosemary in a cup, pour 1 tbs boiling water over them, leave to seep for 5 mins then strain. Add the rosemary and thyme liquid to the bath gel then stir in 10-12 drops of Fern oil. Keep stirring until the smell of Fern hits your nose. Transfer to 200ml plastic bottle, replace bottle cap and it's ready for Uncle Fred.

What about your Mum or Aunt? I'm thinking they'd like the smell of **Rose, Geranium and Neroli** when they're soaking in the tub? Nothing to do other than add 4-5 drops of each oil to your 200ml bottle of ready prepared bath gel. Replace bottle cap, give bottle a gentle shake and you're done.

What about people you don't know well? Everyone loves **Lemon, Lime** and **Orange**. Safe bet. Make that.

Goddess Body Spray. I don't use perfume on my skin. I use body sprays made with essential oils to tune me into nature and uplift my spirit. There are *so* many essential oils you can use in your Goddess body sprays. You can make them to energise or calm, they have super health benefits and smell heavenly.

Women who see the glass as half full and have a positive outlook on life, would probably enjoy body sprays with some of the following essential oils. **Wild Orange, Bergamot, Ylang Ylang, Vetiver, Sandalwood, Geranium, Rose.**

Women who see the glass as half empty and suffer with stress would benefit from a body spray with the following essential oils. **Lavender, Chamomile, Jasmin, Bulgarian Rose.**

I'll tell you how to make a **Geranium, Ylang Ylang** and **Wild Orange** body spray so you see how easy it is. You can then create your own masterpieces using *any* three essential oils of choice from either category.

Just transfer 100ml Rose water into a 100ml glass spray bottle. Add 6 drops Geranium oil, 6 drops Ylang Ylang, and 4 drops Wild Orange oil and a tsp of **vodka.** (the vodka's important because it disperses the essential oils into the rose water). Replace spray cap on bottle, give it a shake and you're ready to make someone feel like a goddess.

Aren't we having fun making these gifts? No stress or strain. No being jostled in the streets by frantic Xmas shoppers - and they cost so little to make, we'll have money left over to treat *ourselves* to something.

With treats in mind, who wouldn't want whipped gingerbread and orange body butter as a gift?

Whipped Gingerbread and Orange Body Butter.

All you need is: A quarter cup **of coconut oil**, half a cup of *****shea butter**, 2 tbs **apricot kernel oil**, oil from 2 **Evening Primrose** capsules, 1 tsp ground **ginger,** half tsp ground **cinnamon**, 8 drops of **Orange oil**.

*Shea butter is difficult to work with when it's rock hard so always melt in a dish over a pan of boiling water before use.

Melt shea butter in a dish over a pan of boiling water, leave to cool slightly then add all your other ingredients. Whip together until you have a smooth consistency.

Leave mixture to nearly harden (it happens fast) then whip again with electric hand mixer, (or egg beater if you don't have one) until it turns fluffy and then transfer to suitably sized pot. Voila. Another great gift. (why not increase quantities and make more using different essential oils?)

And what did I promise you at the beginning of this book? That by the end you'd be whipping up Coconut Souffle Body Cream and Strawberry-Vanilla Mousse Exfoliator with the ease of whipping an egg.

Coconut Souffle Body Cream.

All you need is: 1 cup of melted **Shea Butter**, 2 tbs **Coconut Oil**, 1 tbs **Sweet Almond** oil, 1 tsp **Argan** oil, 1 tsp **Evening Primrose oil**, 10 drops *essential **Coconut Oil.** (*It's different to carrier oil version)

As soon as the shea butter melts, add all ingredients and beat shea butter mixture with an electric hand mixer until it becomes light and fluffy. Add 10 drops essential coconut oil, beat for another ten seconds and you're done.

The least messy way to transfer any recipe into a pot is to spoon the mixture into a small plastic food bag. Twist the top to seal, cut a small hole at the bottom of plastic bag, imagine you are piping a cream cake, pipe mixture into the pot and smooth over.

Strawberry-Vanilla Mousse Exfoliator.

Here's a twist on a face scrub that has a fluffy feel and smells so delicious you'll want to eat it.

All you need are: Quarter cup of melted shea butter, quarter cup of coconut oil, quarter cup of white sugar, 6 drops Strawberry oil, 4 drops Vanilla oil.

Beat all ingredients with an electric hand mixer until mixture fluffs. Transfer to pot, leave to set and it's ready.

Go back through this book and see what else your family or friends might like for Xmas. Put pretty labels on your gifts. Go to town and decorate with sprinkles, sparkles and inspiration.

I have very much enjoyed sharing this journey with you but for now, this is where we part ways. Stay blessed, and don't take life too seriously. The sun shines better on the sunny side.

Printed in Great Britain
by Amazon

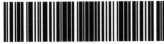